THE CAKE THEORY

THE ROOT CAUSE OF MENTAL ILLNESS AS DISCOVERED BY A PATIENT

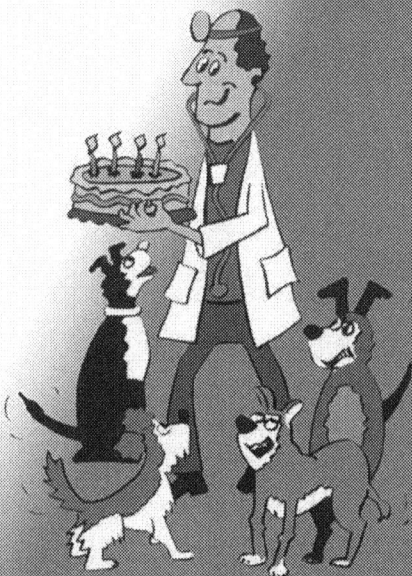

By Alessandro Prian

"One million people commit suicide every year."
The World Health Organisation

Front cover illustration and illustrations of alien, the bowl, ingredients and cooking process by
Mr Frank Canning
(www.frankcanningartist.co.uk). Comic strip illustration by Alessandro Prian.

Published by:
Chipmunkapublishing
PO Box 6872
Brentwood
Essex
CM13 1ZT
United Kingdom

http://www.chipmunkapublishing.com

ISBN 978 1 84747 003 4

Acknowledgements

I'd like to dedicate the following text to Suge Knight and all the artists at the Death Row record label. I'd like to thank them for their music, especially the 'Death Row Greatest Hits' album which really helped me in coming to terms with reality. Listening to their music doesn't inspire me to pick up a gun. I simply enjoy listening to the hearts and minds of people stranded on America's death row.

Contents

1 The Cake Theory

When it comes to mental illness there seems to be no definitive conclusion as to the exact cause. Different books give different opinions and seem to back their theories with evidence even if their evidence is subjective. For example if one were to argue that bad parenting was the root cause of schizophrenia they would offer an example saying 'of the 600 adults assessed with schizophrenia 70% were neglected or mistreated before the age of 6.' However they wont tell you that in a different case study these findings were not reached because this would contradict their **assumption**.

Another book may argue that parenting has nothing to do with it and opt for the genetic cause. Another book will argue it as combination of the two until of course a new study comes along and says neither genetics or parenting was the cause because abnormalities in the brain were discovered and this is the root cause. The psychoanalysts will reject the field of psychiatry and neurology and stick with views laid out by Sigmund Freud.

Having a history of mental illness and being diagnosed with manic depression (which I dispute) I feel it only right that I contribute my own ideas and I've decided to call it "The Cake Theory". This is because in my opinion schizophrenia and other mental disorders have more than one contributory factor and there are a variety of ingredients needed to develop it just as there are a number of ingredients that make up a cake.

2 The History of Mental Illness

In early Egypt mental illness was believed to be caused by environmental factors like loss of status or being made destitute. The treatment involved talking about your problems and turning to religion and faith. It was acceptable to commit suicide at the time. Later the ancient Egyptians changed the theory and decided all illnesses have physical causes. They thought the heart was the root cause of mental illness.

In approximately 500BC when Greek and Roman civilizations began to flourish, philosophers and physicians often conflicted in their opinions regarding the mentally ill. Hippocrates (460-377BC) created the roots of modern medicine and thought mental illness was caused by some kind of internal physical problem like a brain disease. He believed all diseases are caused by an imbalance in the body's four fluids which he referred to as "humors". The four fluids were yellow bile, black bile, blood and phlegm. An imbalance in these fluids was thought to cause mental problems.

Plato (400BC) developed the theory that the soul is driven by 2 forces. He describes these forces in a philosophical sense as being like a charioteer controlling 2 horses. One of the horses is noble and the other is driven by desire. The charioteer finds it difficult to control and balance their opposing impulses. He discuses sexual conflict in man and many people find his work similar to Freud's latter theory of unconscious.

Asclepiades was a Greek doctor who influenced Roman treatments for the mentally ill. He developed cures similar to physiotherapy and concentrated on creating relaxing living environments. He designed a swinging bed and used music to help patients relax. He firmly disapproved of locking up patients and treating them in an inhumane manner. One of Asclepiades followers thought that mania could be treated with alkaline waters which contained high levels of lithium. The Roman treatment for the mentally ill generally involved a pleasant approach which included massage, warm baths, diet, comfortable surroundings and music. They did however sometimes use shocks from electric eels.

As history progressed, the notion that the victim was to blame became the accepted norm. Explanations like evil spirits and moral decline created the stigma that is still evident today. In the 13th century in the United Kingdom one of the first mental institutions was established. The infamous Bedlam was a place where the mentally ill were chained to walls and society conveniently forgot about their existence. Patients were later referred to as 'inmates' and there was no distinction between the mentally ill and the criminally insane. Patients were crowded into dark cells sometimes sleeping five to a mattress near damp floors, firmly chained in position. There was no fresh air or light and they were regularly whipped and beaten. It's important to remember that this was a period when the Church governed and dictated society. This only strengthened the theory that the mentally ill were the work of the devil. Some of the mentally ill were even put to death.

An American colonist referred to the mentally ill as 'lunatics'. This word comes from the word lunar meaning moon because it was thought the moon had something to do with the root cause of mental illness. Methods of treatment involved submerging the patient in iced baths until they lost consciousness, induced vomiting and the notorious bleeding practice. This procedure involved cutting the patient and draining the bad blood however it usually resulted in the death of the individual.

The first mental asylum in America opened in 1769 founded by Benjamin Rush. He also became known as America's first psychiatrist and other asylums were opened all over the country. Rush decided to abolish whips, chains and straitjackets, however he introduced his own method of keeping control of the patient.

The "tranquilizing chair" which can be seen below was his personal favourite and at the time it was considered a lot more humane than being chained to a wall.

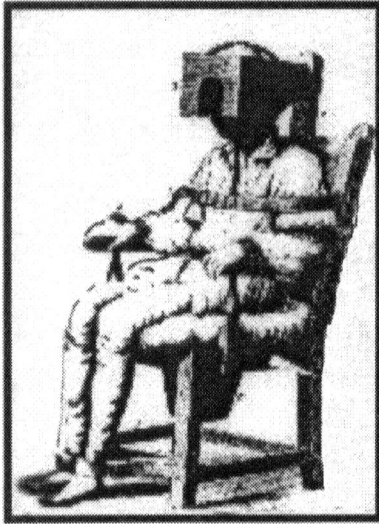

Sigmund Freud (1856–1939) was the founder of the psychoanalysis movement. Freud introduced the theory that patients classified as hysterics might have purely psychological factors contributing to their illness rather than organic brain disease. Freud was born at a time when most of Europe was changing from an agricultural society into an industrialized one. This was an era of new inventions and technological developments and he decided that the mind of a man could be just as complicated and as intricate as a machine. He developed the theory that the mind has many hidden and deep layers which are all governed by the unconscious. He concluded that people with chronic mental illness have a fixation and obsession with the anal region. He believed this fixation originated from a childhood desire of getting pleasure from going to the toilet and a perversion from an infantile age. The mental person's deep dark hidden secret of the unconscious mind.

In the 1930's a new cure for the mentally ill was discovered called lobotomy, and Walter J. Freemen developed the trans-orbital technique. This procedure was performed by sedating the patient and applying quick shocks to the head. One of the eyelids was rolled back and a needle the size of a thin pencil was inserted into the patients head. The device was hammered in to position after which a swinging motion of the needle was created within the patient's skull. Lobotomy became common practice and it was only after the death of many patients that it was abolished. This period also saw a rise in the number of patients undergoing electro convulsive treatment (ECT). Because the level of electricity was so high some patients died or suffered brain damage. In the 1950's the medical profession introduced an anti-psychotic drug called Thorazine for the treatment of the mentally ill. Anti -psychotic medication helped shorten the length of time patients spent in institutions. In fact there was a decline in asylum populations and though patients are no longer physically detained many feel imprisoned within their own minds.

In the United Kingdom ECT treatment is still given however the level of electrical current is much lower. The treatment involves laying a patient on a bed and removing their shoes, watch etc. Present in the room are an anaesthetist (someone who puts you to sleep) a psychiatrist and a nurse. A couple of electrodes are placed on the patients head and he is given injections to relax the muscles and put him to sleep. An electrical current of around 80 volts is given and his muscles begin to twitch. The anaesthetist then passes a tube down his throat to ensure he doesn't choke. Once the doctors have finished the patient is woken up. There are around 130,000 treatments in Britain each year and the most astonishing fact is that nobody knows exactly how it works and there is no conclusive evidence to support its use.

Today people who live in certain countries belonging to Eastern Europe have dreams of coming to the west to better their lives. They hope to one day own a big house with a pool, a fancy car and some even want fame. But where do they keep their mentally ill? In a cage heavily sedated so they don't disturb everybody's dream.

3 Anthropology

Anthropology is the study of human interaction with society and its customs. This is an important issue to discuss since "The Cake" section discusses how a human's environment can affect their mental health. A persons environment is usually dictated by certain ideologies and different ideologies will affect different people differently. Ideology is important to examine because it not only affects the way we view ourselves but also the way we view others. In this section we will only briefly look at anthropology in general terms and draw conclusions relating to mental health in "The Cake" section of the theory.

In the 7th century AD the Islamic faith was founded and Muslim armies were responsible for conquering Mesopotamia, Syria, Palestine, Egypt and Persia. The rapid military and political campaigns were seen by the Muslims as a confirmation that Islam is the best Ideology and cannot be resisted. The Muslims had also conquered the Holy Lands and built "The Dome of The Rock" on top of an important part sacred to Judaism. In the 8th century Muslims tried to attack Constantinople which was the heart of the Eastern Church. The people in Western Europe were predominantly Christians and became worried that Islam would threaten their lifestyle and ideology. In 1095 Pope Urban II gave a public speech and called on people to rescue their fellow Christians who had been conquered by the Muslim armies. He also wanted to regain Jerusalem which was by now under Muslim control for more than 400 years. The crowd shouted "God Wills It" and got ready for battle. Many of the crowd would cut a red piece of cloth into the shape of a cross to wear which became the symbol of the Crusader knights. The Pope promised the people that if they took up arms and thought in the name of God and Christianity they would be forgiven for their sins. The speech by Pope Urban II inaugurated the first Crusade 1095–1099. The Crusaders eventually made it to Jerusalem and much devastation was caused to the city. Muslims and Jews were slaughtered in large numbers and the whole city was stained in human blood. The Crusaders then wrote a letter to the Pope informing him of their successful mission.

A few decades after the first Crusade the Christians began to lose territory. The Turks captured the city of Edessa and killed all its inhabitants. In 1145 Pope Eugenius III decided in favour of another Crusade however his idea was not considered plausible by the nobles. Bernard of Clairvaux was a very powerful figure in the Church and began advocating for the need of a new Crusade. More than 50,000 people participated in France alone and the second Crusade was born (1145-1148). However this Crusade was not very successful and considered a failure because of the lack of military conquests. By the 12th century England and France were at war with each other and unable to maintain control of its Crusader kingdoms in the Holy Land.

The greatest enemy of the Crusades "Saladin" was making progress in Egypt. Saladin managed to defeat Crusader armies and in 1187 captured Jerusalem. The Muslims provoked offence by dragging the Cross of the Holy Sepulcher through the streets and destroying Christian symbols. Saladin had also managed to capture 50 Crusader castles. Pope Gregory VIII called upon people to recapture their lost territory. The three most important Christian figures were Richard the Lionhearted of England, Philip II of France and Frederick Barbarossa of Germany. Once again Muslims were massacred and land was recaptured however were not as successful as the first Crusade.

Most historians believe there were 8 Crusades in total however this doesn't included the Peasants Crusade, Children's Crusade, the Albigensian Crusade etc. Most of the early Crusades were fighting for "forgiveness of sins" and their belief in God and their Christian Ideology.

Even after the Crusades the Muslims tried to impose their beliefs on to others. In the very early stages of the Ottoman Empire, (before they reached their military peak) they saw themselves as "ghazis" warriors of the Muslim faith. In 1389 they attacked Kosovo and imposed Islam which is why you find Muslims in the Balkan region to this day.

Meanwhile in Europe by the 14th and 15th century the Pope had an enormous amount of power and was involved in countless wars predominantly with other Italian states. The Church was involved in corruption and people began to question their wealth as most Popes came from affluent noble families. The people who protested against the Church became known as the "Protestants" and Protestant Churches began to appear all over Europe. One of the reasons that angered the Protestants was the Church selling certificates known as "indulgences". These certificates were confirmation of "forgiveness of sin" and were available to anyone who had money to buy them. In effect the Church became a type of business and Martin Luther was so disgusted that he nailed a list of objections on a church door. His argument was that the only way to be forgiven for sin was through repentance and not by financial means. This event is marked as the beginning of a period known as the "Reformation" and created a division in the Church. Protestants became a threat to traditional Catholicism and wars were thought because of a change in religious ideology. Once again religion was responsible for war, misery and human bloodshed.

The Church remained a dominant force in European society for many years until after the French Revolution. In 1804 Napoleon Bonaparte developed the Napoleonic Code which had a great influence on laws made in Europe and Latin America. Most of the laws in this era were developed from Roman law, medieval systems of religious doctrines. A series of books was developed containing laws which affected the enjoyment of civil rights, divorce, emancipation, marriage settlements, contract limitations etc. The laws passed saw the expulsion of religion governing institutions paving the way for a secular ideology. Most of the laws passed in the Napoleonic Code were based on "common sense".

In the 18th century the United Kingdom became the first country to industrialize its economy. It was only a matter of time before other countries started to industrialize their economy's too. Marxism is a range of theories founded by Karl Marx in the 19th century questioning the industrial revolution and domination of capitalism. Marxism analyses the impact of capitalism on a human beings environment and the inequalities that are produced. The actual theory is complicated and touches on history, economics and philosophy.

Other philosophers belonging to the movement include Hengel, Feuerbach and Kant.

One of the aspects examined was interaction between materialism and ideology. They defined this study as "Dialectical Materialism". Hengel thought that political events, ideas and social groups were all relative to one another and constantly changing. He describes this pattern of change as "dialectic". The change happens when two opposite forces or sets of ideas conflict with each other and then merge in to a third entity. The third entity eventually turns in to a force or set of ideas which meets an opposite force and the process reoccurs resulting in change. Marxism has another concept called "Historical Materialism" which argues that social change happens by human forces and not because of God, destiny or other non human force. This concept also examines how human beings use tools in order to work which are referred to as "forces of production". Different groups of people use different tools and social groups are created based on how they use their tools. The people who decide how other people use their tools are referred to as "relations of production" an example of which would be the government. The combination of these two forces is known as "mode of production". Different modes of production have created different human environments which include a primitive environment, slave environment, feudal environment, capitalist environment and socialist environment.

Marx examines the inequalities arising from capitalism and describes it as being similar to the slave system. Marx predicts that the inequalities in capitalism will create conflict and evolve in to socialism. He sees socialism as a utopian mode of production and when capitalism develops in to socialism it will remain so forever. Marx sees the creation of two groups, the labourer and the capitalist. There is also a third group called the "bourgeoisie" who uphold the values of the capitalist by providing services for example the doctor and teacher. This is described as being similar to the slave environment in the southern United States of the19[th] century when religious beliefs and culture upheld and justified the slave mode of production. In the capitalist system the doctors, teachers etc justify the capitalist mode of production.

In terms of mental health Marxism suggests that economic groups can produce feelings of "alienation" in the labourer. When a person has to sell their potential skill to an employer he becomes a "commodity". The employer has the power to select which "commodity" he prefers by giving job interviews. In a philosophical sense the labourer is no longer human but a tool or object. When a human feels like an object and the only way to survive in a capitalist environment is to become an object the human then begins to feel "alienated". This idea comes from the humanist concept where people are free to govern themselves.

After the Second World War Germany was divided in to four sections. The American, British and French sections were united and called "West Germany" and the Soviet section became known as "East Germany". The West developed a capitalist mode of production and the East became communist. The two different ideologies created a period known as the Cold War. A soviet style communist ideology began to gain power which is why the Americans intervened in Vietnam, in order to stop it spreading. During the Ronald Reagan presidency the communist advance was seen as an "evil force" which threatened the ideals of the West. In fact it was the economic policies of the Soviet Union which led to its collapse and the ending of the Cold war in 1991.

Today many people view the American democratic ideology as being the best just as the Christians believed their ideology was the best during the Crusades. After the atrocities of September 11 2001 a group called the neo conservatives have been gaining power in the American administration. They now have a dream of extending American capitalist ideology throughout the Middle East and beyond. Their vision may backfire and create even more instability in the region.

Even if the neo conservatives did manage to industrialise and impose their ideology not only in the Middle East but the entire planet, you would think they would one day be satisfied. They wouldn't, they would then want to industrialise the moon forgetting what being a human being is all about.

COMIC STRIP

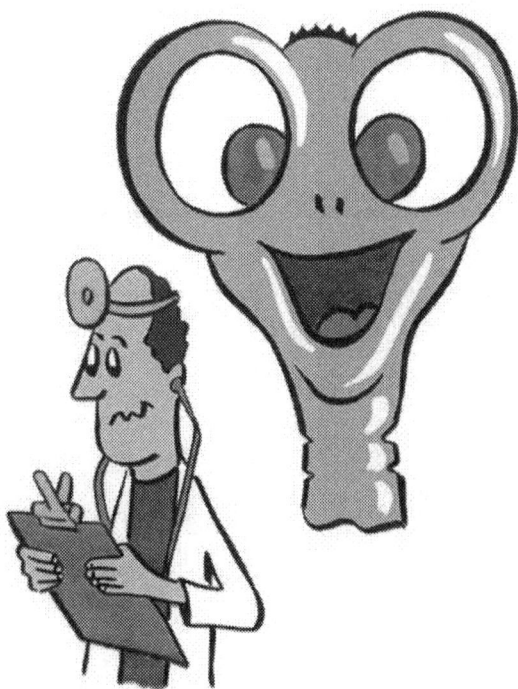

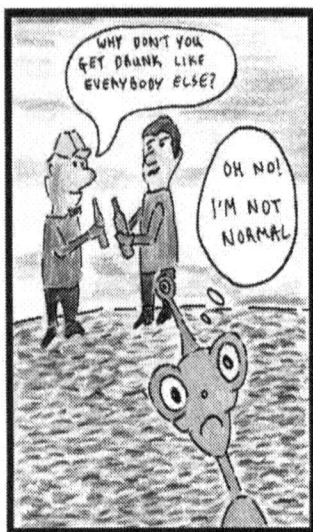

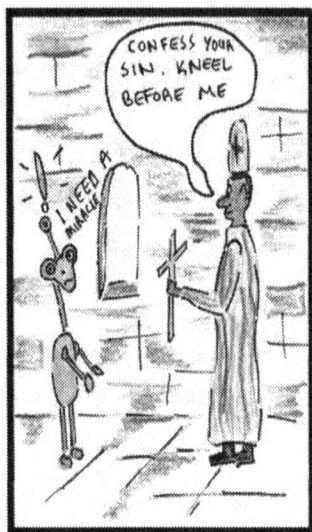

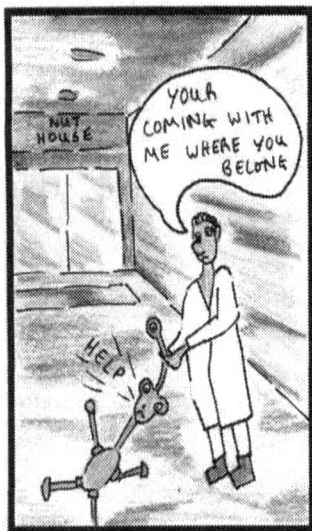

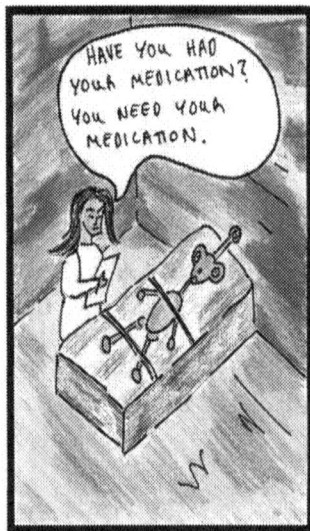

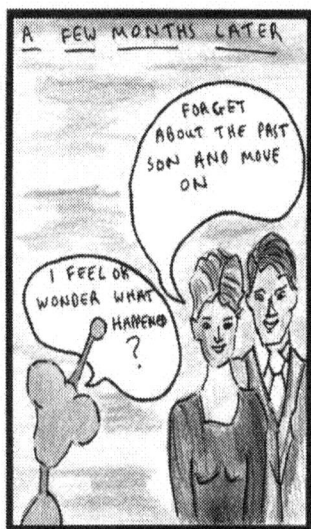

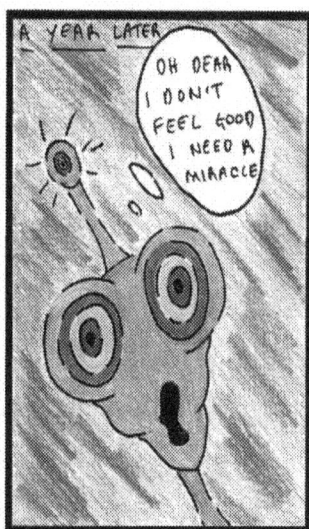

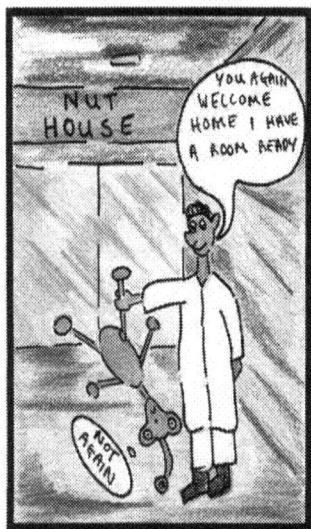

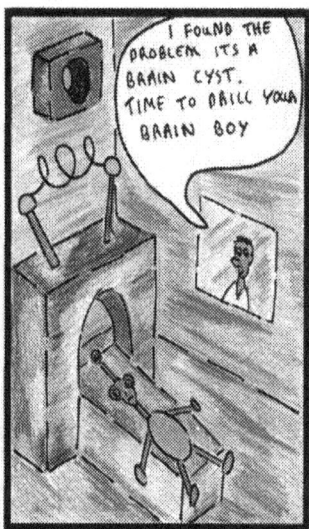

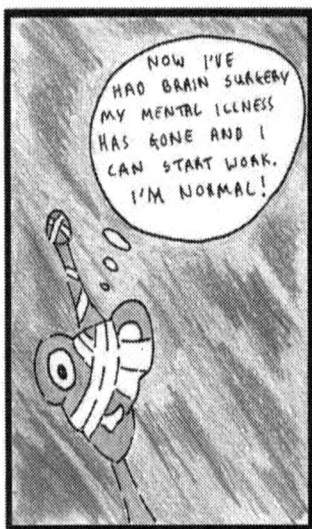

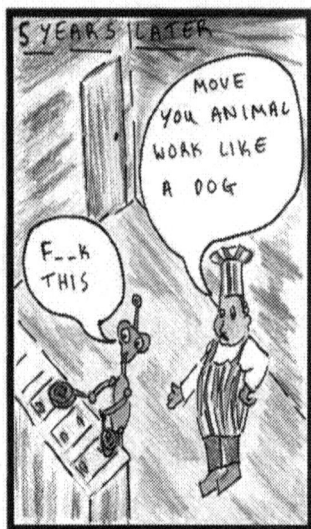

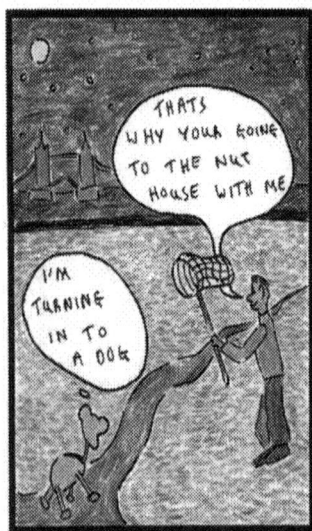

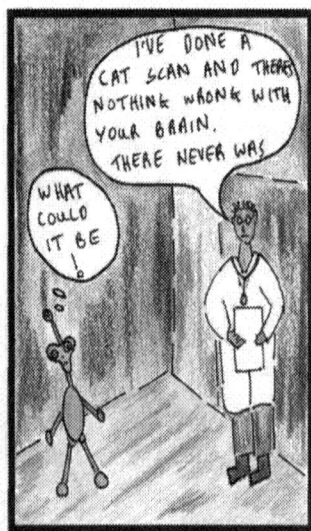

4 My Story

I am of Italian descent born into a moderate catholic household in the United Kingdom. I am now aged 26 and had a normal childhood, and my problems began when I was 16 years of age. My friends would be choosing which college to enrol in, going out every night and getting stoned or drunk but I began to feel like I wasn't part of the group and I didn't fit in. After leaving secondary school I went to college and my anxiety increased. By this time I was a heavy user of marijuana and thought maybe the marijuana was responsible for me feeling uncomfortable. It would leave me feeling drained so I decided anything which could be affecting my mental health should stop and I decided to stop smoking too. By this time my friends were calling me all kinds of unpleasant things and my pain grew strong. My mental pain would appear in bouts and I felt confused and unable to concentrate for a few hours at a time. I asked myself "Why am I feeling like this, what's happening?"

The only logical explanation I could find was the assumption that I was being punished for a sin, my sin being masturbation. I recall watching a television programme where the preacher tells the viewer to hold out his hands and beg for mercy. So there I was in my living room with my arms stretched begging for a miracle. My brain became limited in its ability to concentrate and by now the only book I could comprehend was passages from the Bible. My delusions escalated and I was eventually Sectioned under the Mental Health Act at the age of 18.

In the mental ward I was given a cocktail of drugs and after 28 days released back into the community diagnosed with a breakdown. I began to feel normal and began to embark on a normal way of life. Normal was going to college, getting a good job and eventually joining the housing ladder. After 4 months of taking a series of mind altering drugs I began a six month art course at college. At the end of the course I relapsed and I was taken once again to the mental ward. My delusions as before were of a mystic nature and as before I believed only a divine miracle could save me.

Upon arrival at the hospital I was given blood tests and a CAT scan of my brain, the results of which can be viewed on the following page. The scan revealed a large malformation on my left temporal lobe which the psychiatrists together with the neurosurgeons decided was the cause of my illness. The left side of the brain is associated with personality and emotion. In my deluded mind I didn't want to be operated on and so my parents had to consent on my behalf against my will. The neurosurgeon drilled a hole in my skull and drained the cerebrospinal fluid; however the brain stayed in its abnormal position because the cyst had been there for so long.

The operation was a success and I was sent home after a few days, however I was still suffering from mental delusions and a distorted view of reality. After a few days my mother showed me the x-ray of my brain taken from the CAT scan and it was at that precise moment that I was cured. This was the miracle I had been praying for. "I am normal, this massive arachnoid cyst which is as clear as the blue sky was the cause of my problems." (Image flipped vertically)

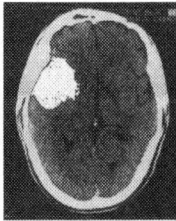

A few months after the operation my family invited the head psychiatrist who discovered the brain cyst to my house for a thank you dinner. At the dinner the psychiatrist assured my family that I would never again set foot in to a mental ward because my illness had been cured. My family then congratulated and applauded the psychiatrist for her marvellous work in discovering the root cause of my mental illness.

TEST RESULTS

REQUESTED BY PSYCHIATRIC DEPARTMENT

ECG -   Sinus tachicardia - frequency 110 otherwise within normal limits.

Blood Tests -   FBC – normal, except Platelets – 135,000 mm3, Reticolocytes 1.3%. U&E, Ca++, Phosph, Creatinine, B.S, LFT, GGT, LDH HBDH, Amylase, Lipids, protein, electrophoresis, uric acid, Cholinesterase, TSH, T3, T4 – all normal values.
CPK : 994 U/L (20-180). Blood Group – AB RH POS. Iron – 42mcg/dl (60-140) Seric Feritim, PTT, APTT all normal.

HBs Abs:	negative
HBs Ag:	negative
HBc Abs:	negative
VDRL:	negative
TPHA:	negative

CAT Scan -   Scan of head, section of 5mm thickness reveals presence of a coarse large area of hypodensity which occupies the left side of the middle cranial fossa.

MRI Scan -   Images obtained with SE technique in T1 on sagital sections in DP and T2 on axial sections, in Flair technique on coronal sections. This test confirms the Cat scan.

EEG -   Alpha activity almost absent. Beta activity of medium amplitude and increased frequence dominant on the frontal regions and parieto – temporal on both hemispheres. Rare Theta waves bilaterally. No alterations during HP and SLI. Absence of epileptiform abnormalities and slow pathological waves.

X-Ray-   Chest X – Ray : no parenchimal active focal alteration. No pleural effusion. Cardiomediastinic image within normal limits.

I then began a period of reflection and reached a strong conviction that all people with mental illness have an organic cause for example a tumour, chemical imbalance etc. I began to think I was the lucky one because I was not mentally ill anymore. This also led me to believe that if it wasn't for my brain operation I would probably still be in the mental ward. I developed a strong appreciation for technology and science because if it wasn't for them, who knows what would have happened to me. I became interested in technology and thought how tremendously beneficial it is for society.

A year passed after the operation and I went to university studying a design orientated course. I felt reasonably comfortable because on a degree course you're left to your own devices and I graduated after 3 years. I thought I could now do any job I wished because the cyst was drained and my mental illness had gone. At the time a bit of a cynic, I never expected to get a job in my chosen field because this was difficult, however lots of people have this problem. I began to suffer from a pain in the ass which I assumed was haemorrhoids though a doctor had never confirmed this. To me it was logical as there was a history of haemorrhoids in the family and I used suppositories as I thought this would help.

I found a job working in an estate agent which was

initially quite enjoyable as I was meeting people and arranging appointments. It was quite difficult getting a sale and it was a hectic environment. After 3 months my haemorrhoids were very discomforting and on one evening I developed a feeling of being light headed and wanting to lie in a dark room. I had a powerful headache and had to remain in the dark for hours. This had never happened before and I was quiet worried. I called in sick at work and then went to the doctor and expressed my concerns that it could be my brain cyst but was assured it was probably a migraine due to stress. I told the doctor that may very well be the case but it might be something else. I explained to the doctor all I had done was sit in an office, make a few calls and meet a client, something a 15 year old could do. I insisted on a blood test and the doctor complied. After a couple of days the blood test results proved negative.

The estate agent I worked for relocated and I found myself out of work. I began to look for another job and saw an advert for a chef which I thought could be fun as I had worked in restaurants before. I thought I could work as a chef for a year, get some money and then progress in a different career. Initially working in the kitchen seemed enjoyable, however after a few weeks the hours were increased and so was the work load. On more than one occasion I was working on the pasta section cooking several dishes simultaneously for 3 hours after which big bowls of soup and then I even had to clean up. I knew I was being exploited so I told the manager and was promised things would improve. At this point my haemorrhoids were really painful and decided as embarrassing as it may be I should visit a doctor. I visited my GP and was later referred to a specialist. By now my sex life with girl's was affected because it was like drinking a glass of wine with a sore throat.

I looked on the internet for different ways of removing haemorrhoids and decided to opt for the elastic band treatment. The day came and I went to the doctor to be examined and upon examination the doctor said something about not seeing anything wrong and prescribed me an ointment. I was shocked, so I took the prescription and walked out without saying goodbye. I said to myself "What kind of a doctor is he? He couldn't see any haemorrhoids and he used a machine! Looks like I'll have to go to another doctor". Embarrassed at the prospect of being examined again I decided maybe I had misunderstood what he said so I wrote him a letter thanking him for his time and asked if he could kindly put my diagnosis in writing.

I went back to work as a chef and my working conditions deteriorated even more. On one particular day, three of my work colleagues who were waiters told me that they were getting paid more money than I was for half of the hours I worked. I really flipped and threw my chef's jacket on the floor and told the manager what to do with the pasta. By now I was fuming so I went home and upon entering my house I found a letter on the door mat which can be viewed on the following page. I picked it up and read it and couldn't believe it. It was the doctor confirming that he couldn't find any haemorrhoids, however he went further to say he couldn't find anything wrong with me. This really threw me off the edge. "Has this doctor taken me for a pervert, maybe he thinks I get my kicks this way"? I threw the letter on the floor and began to wander the streets of London trying to find somewhere that made sense, like a lost dog trying to understand his life. I began to feel high as if I had taken cocaine or heroin though as I've never taken these drugs I couldn't be sure.

I wandered the streets all night searching, until my energy was drained and I fell to the ground. I phoned for an ambulance but in my mental state the operator thought I was a hoax caller. I then reversed the charges and phoned home, told my sister the name of the street I was in and she came to pick me up. When she arrived my sister phoned for an ambulance and I was taken to hospital.

When I arrived at the hospital my body started to shake violently and I was placed in a dark room for 10 minutes where I cooled down. My sister explained to the nurse that my mental illness was caused by a brain cyst and I needed to undergo a CAT scan. Once again my brain was put under the microscope so to speak in order to verify if the cyst needed operating on. I began to think of the prospect of undergoing surgery and it wasn't a pleasant thought.

The radiologist then entered the room holding a copy of the CAT scan, you can see it below.

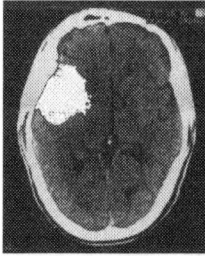

He said "There's no need to operate" so I told him to open his eyes because there must be something wrong. The radiologist then said "This type of cyst is usually an incidental finding and neurosurgeons rarely operate unless there is internal bleeding. He went on to say "Furthermore had you presented yourself with this kind of cyst when you were mentally unstable 5 years ago I would not have operated on you then". This was all too much for me to take in. One doctor was telling me I never had haemorrhoids in my backside when it was clearly hurting and this one was telling me a cyst never caused my problems when 5 years ago I was told it was. No doubt I had a fit and was sectioned under the Mental Health Act and left only with a puzzle. What caused My mental illness?

North Middlesex University Hospital NHS
NHS TRUST

Colorectal Unit
Consultants
Mr Luke Meleagros MD FRCS
Mr Romi Navaratnam MSc MS FRCS

Macmillan colorectal nurse specialist
Sue Williams RGN/NMB216, ENB998, ENB237
Specialist registrar
Mr cheuk Bong Tang BSc(Hons), MSc, MS, FRCS(Ed.)

Sterling Way
London N18 1QX
Direct Line 020 8887 2241
Direct Fax 020 8887 2362

Secretary. Ruth Sims BSc(Hons)
E-mail ruth.sims@nmh.nhs.uk

NHS No : ▓▓▓▓▓
Typed : 16.5.03

Clinic: 13.5.03
Re : ▓▓▓▓▓▓▓

Dear Alessandro Prian

I enclose a copy of my letter to your GP following your recent consultation. As you can see when I examined you I did not find any evidence of haemorrhoids.

....

Many thanks for referring this young man. His symptom is anal pain for the past year. It is painful all the time and not particularly at defecation. The bowel habit is regular without constipation. There is no rectal bleeding.

Rectal examination was normal. There was no evidence of fissure or sphincter spasm. Sigmoidoscopy to 15cm was normal. Proctoscopy did not reveal any piles.

I explained to him that there is no evidence of first degree piles or any other pathology to account for his symptoms. He is rather dissatisfied because he was keen on an answer and a cure. I prescribed GTN ointment on the assumption that the pain relates to increased muscular activity in the sphincters. I will see him in 3 months.

Best wishes,

Yours sincerely

▓▓▓▓▓▓

Consultant surgeon

THE
BOWL

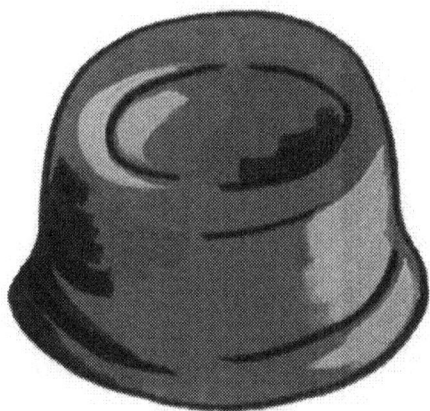

5 The Human Experience

Before you make a cake you need a bowl and this is the same in mental illness. The bowl in mental illness is one's initial perception of reality. The big mistake all people with mental illness make is that they look around their environment and compare themselves to their friends or immediate surroundings. In doing so you have created the Bowl.

In my case when I was 16 my friends would be getting their driving licences, losing their virginity and going to college. To me this was normal, every one does it and I began to feel a different kind of 'normal' because I didn't really want to go to the pub every night and get drunk and I never really wanted a driving licence therefore I began to say "There's something wrong with me". This created the Bowl. Something that never occurred to me was that in my year at school there were over 200 students and not all of them were going out every night.

To really be realistic the mental person must be fully aware of the bowl, (their surrounding environment and how much it can affect them). This is not done by closing your eyes and wishing for something different, it is done by opening your eyes and looking at the whole human condition and the state of being a human being. I'll begin by giving you an analogy with a tree.

A tree is a tree, there it is blowing in the wind tall and strong. Or is it? It seems in the western world trees fall into two distinct categories. They are known as endogens and exogenous. The endogens grow both longitudinally and diametrically however the exogenous grows diametrically with a new layer being formed each year.

Of the exogenous type they fall into another two categories being deciduous and the conifer. The deciduous also known as hardwood sheds its leaves annually and the conifer also known as softwood retains its leaves all year round. Both of them are trees, neither is better than the other, both are equal. Or are they? Well it seems if we take wood and use it for flooring the hardwood is more durable than the soft. It's better, it lasts longer and the colours are generally nicer. The tree is no longer equal but the environment that we have chosen to place it in has made one better than the other.

A man is a man or is he? If there are two, then both remain men, neither one is better than the other, both are equal. Or are they? It seems they also fall into two distinct categories, the extrovert and the introvert. The extrovert is more concerned with their immediate external reality than with inner feelings and the introvert is more concerned with his own thoughts and feelings. It seems in the western world we are encouraged to become more like the extrovert from a young age. We are brainwashed into thinking that the extrovert is more superior. The extrovert succeeds in business "the entrepreneur" progresses and is confident he will make it in life and we praise and admire him. The classical line from a father is "son one day you'll make something of yourself." In other words the only way to become a complete man would be to become a manager or boss.

The characterisation has been extended and not only is there an introvert and an extrovert but there is a secure person and an insecure person. Because 50 % of man is introvert we've extended the characterisation process even further. A few examples are personality disorder, multiple personality disorder, narcissism, manic depression, schizophrenia etc. It now seems the characterization process is verging on the ridiculous and soon we will see the "lawnmower syndrome" where the individual takes on the personality of a gardener and mows the grass three times a month instead of the recommended once a month.

It seems that man is no longer equal. One is better

than the other; however let us go back to the tree analogy.

We came to the conclusion before that hardwood is better than softwood. It's strong, it's more durable. We could use the softwood as a flooring material but it is only chosen because it's cheaper, because hardwood is better, or is it?

Well, if we were to use the tree for structural purposes for example the frame of a house, the softwood is better. The properties of the softwood make it more able to work in this environment as it is less rigid and more flexible etc. The tables have turned and the softwood is better and superior.

Let us turn the tables on modern day life in the western world by letting the introverts run and dictate society. We can do this by using empathy and I have done this by creating a fictitious Newspaper which can be viewed on the following pages.

THE DAILY NEWS

THE LEADERSHIP SYNDROME

This is a condition where the leader becomes indulged in his own grandiose fantasy. It seems the root cause of this syndrome or illness has yet to be discovered but it could be due to a brain malformation or childhood upbringing. It does seem confidence plays a crucial role because when the individual is confident he loses sight of the people around him. It seems that confidence is not enough and the individual then begins the abnormal state of leadership. In his deluded mind he hungers the need for superiority and many analysts believe this was lack of love as a child. The lack of love could lead him to believe that leadership will fill a hole in the void in his personality and it seems the more he gets, the more he wants, eventually turning into megalomania and the empire syndrome.

Let us look at a classical example from a secondary school textbook in the national curriculum. This is how it reads "Alexander the Great, a brilliant young general, created the largest empire the world has ever seen, a gifted young leader who inspired loyalty from his troops." But is he brilliant and great? Or is he a murderer who managed to convince the extroverts. There are still statues of Alexander, stone representations of what he really was, a man with a heart of stone. More than 2000 years later this syndrome is still evident. In 1935 Mussolini decided to invade Abyssinia in Africa. The Italian dictator stood in Piazza Venezia (Rome) and announced to a crowd of 400 000 extroverts that Italy had an empire. The only reason he did this was because he had "a dream". A dream or a maniac lost in his own interpretations of reality. Why didn't anyone put this lunatic in an asylum? Today nothing much has changed. For the Queens Jubilee celebration the extroverts stood outside Buckingham Palace and sang "Rule Britannia, Britannia rules the waves."

If the world is divided in two, if there is night and day, positive and negative then who could be the exact opposite of the leader. Who could be the exact opposite of Alexander the Great, both equally as blind, both lost in their own deluded mind. Who other than our dear friend Mr. Schizophrenia, a man with a heart in pain and suffering.

THE CONFIDENCE SYNDROME
(Personality Disorder)

Introverts have been trying to root out confidence in the work place. Confident people are unaware how harmful their actions can be to others and employers are now trying to stamp out confidence in the work place. In a recent case study of 2000 employees it was found that 9 times out of 10 the confident person was responsible for spreading vicious office rumours and was generally more malicious.

The root cause of confidence has yet to be discovered but valium has been shown to be a good drug to cure this illness. Shy people seem to be better equipped in the work place; they get on with their work and meet targets. Employers have decided to conduct aptitude tests before a job is given in order to stamp out confidence in the work place.

JOB SECTION

JOB! JOB! JOB!

Shy person wanted to work in an office environment
Someone polite who enjoys working on
their own initiative
ONLY SHY PEOPLE APPLY

LONER REQUIRED

LONER REQUIRED TO WORK IN A COMPANY
THAT HAS FALLING SALES - ARE YOU ABLE TO
COME UP WITH THE SOLUTION?
ARE YOU THE LONER WE'RE WAITING FOR?
STARTING SALARY 40 THOUSAND A
YEAR PLUS COMPANY CAR

PROBLEM PAGE

Question = Dear Agony Aunt. I've been out of work
for some time and every time I go for an interview it's
the same story "I'm too confident". I know being
confident is a bad thing but I really would like a job.
I've tried pretending by avoiding eye contact and
looking on the floor but they seem to suss me out. Can
you help?

Answer = You said in your letter that you've tried valium and other drugs to calm you down however have you ever considered a psychologist? It could be a deep rooted problem. A recent case study revealed that lack of affection in a person's childhood could contribute towards such problems. Let me know how it goes.

Question = Dear Agony Aunt. I'm 16 years old and I don't fit in at school. Everybody likes staying indoors and listening to music or playing computer games. I know I'm only suppose to go clubbing every blue moon or on special occasions but I find I really want to go every week. I am a nice person, please help.

Answer = You could try cognitive therapy. I see you've accepted that you're nice and this is the classical sign that we see in the beginning stages of the confidence syndrome. So rather than saying "I'm a nice person" try saying "I'm going to make an effort with my fellow students". I enclose some addresses; let me know how you get on.

ADVERT SECTION

Are you over confident?
Do you have a bubbly personality which is irritating
and insensitive?
HYPNOTHERAPY AVAILABLE TO
REVERSE YOUR CONDITION
MAKE THE CHANGE YOU'VE ALWAYS WANTED

End of Newspaper Section

Some members of society are aware of these inequalities and try to get in touch with the human experience by going to a naturist park. This is an environment where everybody is naked and nobody is judged in any way. However the extroverts are unable to see this and say "bunch of perverts, lets go to the pub".

The UK has deemed the hyperactive male as having a problem. In the UK only 2% of the work force is employed in agriculture. Had this man been born in the Philippines where 45% of the population are employed in agriculture, would he have had a problem? Not only would he not have had a problem but the extroverts would all have been jealous of his strength.

We've been brainwashed into thinking a prostitute is scum, but its ok to go out on a Saturday night, tell a girl its love at first sight when all he wants is a f***. There's actually a book published called "They F*** You Up" where the author has described a mental person as being "a f***ed up person". But am I? I feel perfectly fine, I like time alone, swimming, listening to music and getting laid every now and again.

In an agricultural society you could be made to feel different if mum tells you "why can't you be like your brother and go to an industrialised country to send money home". In the school playground everybody likes the bully and the victim acquires a bowl. If people are made to believe they have sinned in a catholic system, someone acquires a bowl.

During the Second World War Hitler managed to convince people that the Jews were "f***ed up people". Using his SS symbol he created a religion and set of values where he convinced the population that the Jewish man is a greedy scum bag and is the cause of society's problems. In 1935 the Jews lost their citizenship and could no longer marry another German. They were expelled from schools and libraries and could no longer use the telephone or open a business. They were formally declared the lowest of the low by the state. In effect when the Jews were rounded up and sent to the concentration camps people no longer saw a fellow human being, but saw someone who is "not equal". However the Jewish man didn't think "oh yes you're right I'm the scum of society". He never said "Jewish blood is different that's why were scum". He never said "we've got an abnormal brain that's why were f***ed up". So why do the mentally ill believe everything were told? Why do we believe them when the extroverts say being shy is a personality disorder? Why do we believe it when Mother F***ers deem us unequal? Why do we care?

These people have a habit of drawing their inspiration

from the animal kingdom. Can you believe they actually study the behaviour of a rat and then compare it to a man? They conveniently say "survival of the fittest" because the environment they have created works for them. I really did think we were so much more than a bunch of animals.

INGREDIENTS

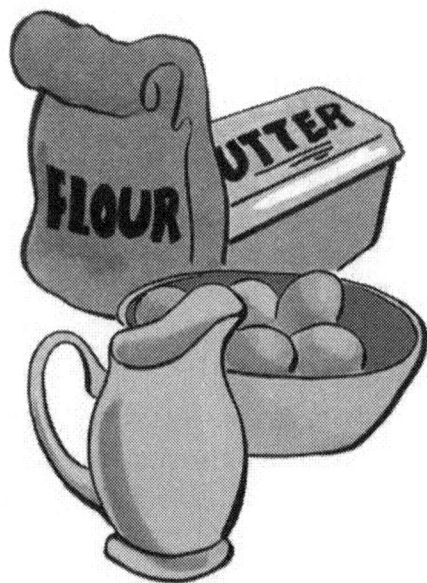

6 Butter & Sugar / Stress & IBS

Now we have our bowl we need to add some melted butter with sugar. In the mental man this is his perception of reality with stress and IBS. First we must look at what stress and irritable bowel syndrome actually are.

Stress is an interference that disrupts a person's mental and physical well-being. Stress may be experienced in response to a range of physical and emotional factors. There are cases of stress being caused by physical illness however the vast majority of cases are provoked by a human being's environment. Some people will argue that a situation provokes stress. This is true however it's important to remember that a situation always occurs in an environment and different environments will have different situations.

As we saw in the opening section "The History of Mental illness" there has been mental illness in every society. This is because different people respond differently to different environments. In my case, at the adolescent stage, the stress of peer pressure and surviving in the western world was overwhelming however it's quite possible a different environment wouldn't have provoked such disastrous consequences.

For example if a university professor was born in one of the many agricultural societies on our planet where books are scarce it's possible this environment would make him lose his sanity as reading and gathering information is vital for his mental well being. Somebody who is good at multitasking in an office environment may have the same problem because in agricultural countries there are few offices and this skill is not required.

Some people in an agricultural society find the stress of not having enough food to feed their family overwhelming and this could drive them insane. However someone who became insane in an industrial society where food is plentiful may have reacted differently if he were born in an agricultural society with little food. It's possible the scarcity of food and less complicated environment could improve his mental health as a survival instinct is aroused and he reacts differently. In the western world some people have a hunger for fame. They want the attention and glamour associated with this way of life. However being famous is one of the most artificial environments known to man. It's not normal to have paparazzi chasing you every time you leave your house and have your every movement under scrutiny. In fact most people would find this environment very hostile and the invasion of privacy could drive them to lose their sanity.

There is of course evidence to support this theory which is dismissed by the psychiatric profession. This is probably because the psychiatrist functions best is a modern environment and expects everybody else to do so. The evidence suggests that in relation to the social classes, mental illness is twice as common among the poor. Mental illness is also three times more likely to occur in American Afro-Caribbean's and 16 times more common in children of West Indian immigrants to Britain. This evidence also contradicts the genetic argument for mental illness because when the relatives of the immigrant schizophrenics from the same family living in the West Indies were studied the rates of mental illness were much lower in their native homeland.

Now we know what causes stress we need to know what happens to our body when placed in a stressful environment. To do this we will first look at the central nervous system which comprises of the brain and spinal cord connected to all other organs in the body. The nerves which connect the organs and muscles to the spinal cord carry messages telling them how to react. There are various systems which control these organs in the body. A human being has a lot of control over the voluntary nervous system. This is the system which allows you to control your muscle movement for example the lifting of a heavy object.

There is however an involuntary or autonomic nervous system which is a lot less easy to control. This also consists of a network of fibres that connects to the central nervous system. This system is responsible for breathing, heartbeat, blood pressure, blinking etc. Although the involuntary system is invaluable, the lack of control can cause problems.

The illustration below will make this easier to understand.

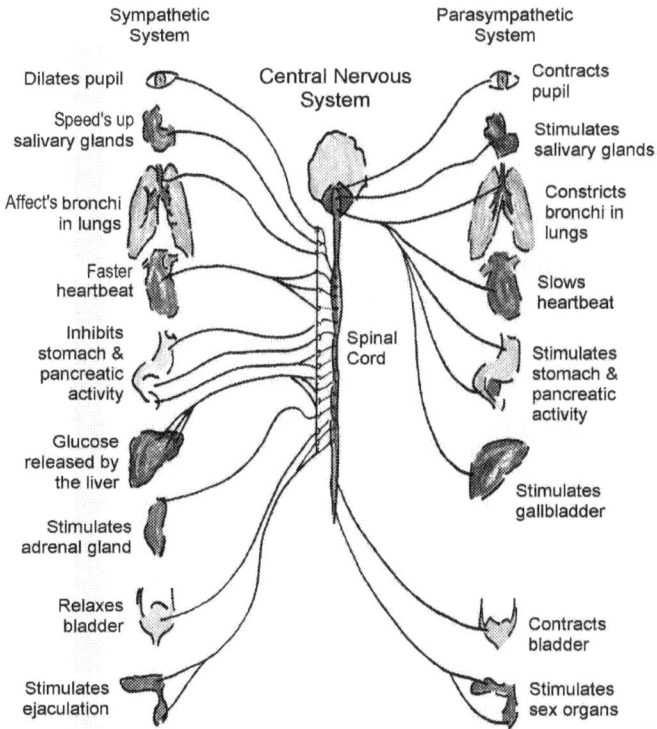

Sympathetic System

Parasympathetic System

Central Nervous System

Dilates pupil

Speed's up salivary glands

Affect's bronchi in lungs

Faster heartbeat

Inhibits stomach & pancreatic activity

Glucose released by the liver

Stimulates adrenal gland

Relaxes bladder

Stimulates ejaculation

Contracts pupil

Stimulates salivary glands

Constricts bronchi in lungs

Slows heartbeat

Spinal Cord

Stimulates stomach & pancreatic activity

Stimulates gallbladder

Contracts bladder

Stimulates sex organs

The involuntary nervous system falls in to two categories known as the sympathetic on the left of the illustration and the parasympathetic system on the right. When a human being is placed in an environment he finds uncomfortable the sympathetic system responds by stimulating certain organs, for example the heart, which in turn increases heart rate. Other organs like the adrenal glands (on top of the kidneys) release chemicals like adrenaline. There may be an increase in muscular activity, less blood going to the stomach and breathing may increase. When the person is taken out of the environment which has provoked these biochemical reactions the parasympathetic nervous system is activated. This system helps the body to return to its normal function and decreases the heart rate etc.

Because the human body is extremely complicated there is also another system which reacts to stress. This is known as the hypothalamic-pituitary-adrenal pathway and is not demonstrated on the illustration. When faced with stress the hypothalamus (the region of the brain controlling body temperature, thirst, hunger etc) signals a small gland at the base of the brain called the pituitary gland. The body's "major stress hormone" is released which then stimulates the adrenal glands provoking the release of cortisol.

At a certain level all these bodily changes can disrupt

a person's ability to cope and can lead to physical symptoms like headache, migraines, panic attacks, anxiety, irritable bowel syndrome etc. However because we are making a specific cake we will only need to look more closely at the latter.

Irritable Bowel Syndrome

This is a biochemical reaction in the body triggered by stress which can result in a physical irritation or pain in the ass. This condition is usually diagnosed when X – Rays and other tests fail to show any abnormalities. IBS is not usually diagnosed by a medical practitioner because the symptoms could be caused by something else.

The condition usually occurs in adolescences or early adulthood because most people find this period very stressful. As discussed in the stress section the body has many organs which react when faced with stress, it seems the bowel is no different to any other organ in the human body.

Going back to my life story after graduating from university and starting work I had a pain which I thought was haemorrhoids. If hypothetically the doctor had found by coincidence haemorrhoids upon examination, I would have been convinced beyond a reasonable doubt that this was the cause of my problem. There would be nothing anyone could ever say or do that would have convinced me otherwise. However I had to accept that nothing was found. But if nothing was found what was the cause? It seems the stress of work provoked a bio chemical reaction in my body which caused an involuntary muscular contraction. How could a simple task like going to an office and making a few phone calls, something that even a 15 year old could do, cause such a reaction? I began to reflect and I do remember that at the age of 16 the stress of school and peer pressure may have provoked a reaction back then but because I was ignorant and had other worries at the time, I never knew what to think. Why didn't anyone come along to my school and explain the causes of stress and how they affect people when I was 14? Why was it left for me to figure out? I was left to feel like an alien.

It really is a scandal. After coming to this realization perhaps the radiologist was correct when I had my last breakdown. Perhaps the cyst had nothing to do with my mental illness and there was no need to operate the second time I was unwell. In retrospect the second time I was unwell after the brain surgery I really only became cured when I saw the CAT scan. The reason I became cured was because I could have taken my scan to my friends and said "Look this is why I was unwell" and I would have been accepted in the community (the placebo effect).

For arguments sake had I not been operated on the second time I was unwell and there was no cyst, I wouldn't have been able to go back to my friends or relatives to get sympathy for my anguish. I wouldn't have been able to get any sympathy because society has deemed the mental person as being the lowest of the low. It's no good pretending otherwise because my fellow human beings have decided this.

It seems the psychiatrists and neurosurgeons looked at my case and saw I was manifesting the classical signs of chronic non-responsive mental illness. They knew if I wasn't to be operated on I would probably live the rest of my life believing a sin was the cause of my illness. In effect they unintentionally tricked me in to believing my mental illness was caused by a brain cyst the same way the Church tricked me in to believing my illness was caused by a sin. I say this also because all the evidence supports the notion that an arachnoid cyst is an incidental finding and should be left alone. Looking through my medical notes the cyst was not under pressure and there was no internal bleeding. It seems another case of assumption on the doctor's part. For those who insist that the cyst must have affected my mental health because they see life only in black and white I have enclosed evidence from a brain surgeon which can be viewed on the following page.

As you can see it seems I have to be thankful for having major brain surgery when I never really needed it in the first place. I say this because had the neurosurgeon not operated I would have been led to believe that a sin or something in my childhood contributed to my mental problems. I would probably now be in a tremendous amount of mental pain whilst being eaten alive by the human vulture also known as 'the psychologist'.

This theory could also be applicable to people who undergo ECT therapy. If there is a belief by the patient and his family that the treatment will be of benefit it could cure him. The whole theatrical procedure could convince the patient that an electrical current in the brain could be of help, it's rather like a priest performing an exorcism in a society governed by the Church. In a secular society the miracle cure is performed by the doctor but in both scenarios the procedure is pointless, unless of course you manage to convince the patient. Just as I was given brain surgery against my will some people are given ECT treatment without their consent when sectioned under the Mental Health Act. It really is a terrible shame.

Now that we have looked at stress as well as the reactions it can provoke, we shall look at a few ways in helping you to deal with stress. I have come up with a few helpful tips to improve your mental health.

• Many people have mental health problems so don't feel embarrassed. Anyone who thinks less of you because you've had mental health issues isn't worth your time or knowing in the first place.

• Be aware how much your surrounding environment can affect you and try to find environments that work for you within the parameters of modern day life. An example would be stay clear of places you find stressful and try to find environments you feel comfortable in.

• Don't value yourself on material wealth or think less of yourself because you don't own a house or luxury car. The important thing in life is to feel like a million dollars not necessarily to have a million dollars in your bank account. If you have your sanity and peace of mind then you are rich enough.

• Human contact is important to relieve stress. You may find it useful to join the Mind Social Club where you can meet people who have had similar experiences making you feel less alien.

• Try to exercise even if it's in the privacy of your own home. Exercise helps the muscles to relax and helps relieve stress.

• If you find it difficult getting to sleep at night buy yourself a small pocket size radio and listen to some of the talk radio programmes. This will keep your mind from thinking to much and help you fall asleep.

• You could try relaxation exercises. These involve breathing in slowly whilst tensing individual muscles of your body helping you to relax.

██████████ **FRCS.FRCPCH**
Consultant Paediatric Neurosurgeon

Dept. of Neurosurgery,
The Radcliffe Infirmary
Woodstock Rd,
Oxford OX2 6HE.

I am ██████████ date of birth 10th May 1954. I am a registered

medical practitioner and I hold the degree of Bachelor of Medicine and

Bachelor of Surgery. I am a Fellow of the Royal College of Surgeons, a

Fellow of the Royal College of Paediatrics and Child Health and I am

on the Specialist Register for Neurosurgery.

I have been in full time medical practice since 1977, full time

neurosurgical practice since 1981 and have been in continuous

employment as a Consultant Neurosurgeon since 1987. I am

currently employed as a Consultant Paediatric Neurosurgeon to the

Oxford Radcliffe Hospitals NHS Trust.

<u>Opinion</u>

Alessandro Prian has an arachnoid cyst. This is a collection of

cerebrospinal fluid which will have been present since birth.

Temporal fossa cysts are associated with hypoplasia of the temporal

lobe and they rarely cause significant cerebral compression. In those

where cerebral compression is significant, their presentation can

include headache, developmental delay and seizures.

The vast majority of arachnoid cysts remain totally asymptomatic and are undetectable, except by brain scanning. Many are discovered when patients are investigated for a condition which turns out to be unrelated to the arachnoid cyst. These commonly include non-specific headaches and following minor head trauma. Whenever they are detected they cause considerable anxiety, both in patients and non-specialist medical staff, and it is often assumed by both, especially when there has been headache or other non-specific neurological symptoms, that they must be linked.

I believe this is what has occurred in Alessandro's case. I have never come across an arachnoid cyst causing severe mental illness. I have consulted six major textbooks of neurosurgery and two of neurology, and in none of them can I find acute mental illness described as a presentation of arachnoid cyst. I have also performed a computerised literature search and the two conditions have not been described together.

My neurosurgical colleague indicated in one of his letters that he could not understand the reasons for exploring the cyst surgically. I agree with him. Had Alessandro presented to me I would not have operated.

My opinion, therefore, is that Alessandro's arachnoid cyst was an incidental finding which had no bearing whatsoever on his mental illness.

7 Egg & Flour / SEX positive & negative

During the reign of Imperial Rome men with a lust for power hid behind the symbol of the sword. The empire grew strong and was fuelled by dreams of wealth, splendour and grandeur. The Arch of Constantine in 315AD marks the end of the empire. Constantine took two decisions ending Rome's historic rule. Firstly he allowed freedom of worship to the Christians and secondly he ended the empire as treachery was present. The ruins of Rome were soon covered in vines and forgotten and a new more perverse empire was born. The Church. Men with a lust for power no longer hid behind the symbol of the sword but could now hide behind the symbol of the Cross.

Going back to my life story you will recall I was convinced that masturbation was the cause of my problem and this was my sin. However had I been told that in 1231 Pope Gregory the 9th established the Papal Inquisition where anyone who questioned the Church was put to death, had I known that Dominican Tomas de Torquemada killed thousands that were against the church in the 15th century, and had I known that it was only as recently as 200 years ago that it stopped, would I have felt that a sin was the cause of my mental illness? Had I known the priest says "sins of the flesh", and when the Church service is over he has sex with a child; if I knew then I would have had a different bowl and I wouldn't have been waiting for a miracle. The mental man does not have a conscience which is any different to anyone else except when led to believe so.

In today's secular society the priest's confessional chamber has been replaced by the psychologist's office and the sin has been replaced with a secret. I'm afraid there is no such thing as the unconscious mind which governs our actions. This is just a fantasy created in the psychologist's office, just as a perverted sin was a fantasy created by the Church. While the patient sits and talks about their childhood the psychologist gets her mortgage, luxury car and holiday paid for. The patient gets nothing.

However, sex does play a part and I have come up with the following. The body contains a certain amount of negative and positive electrical energy, in the brain it is measured with an EEG machine. To understand this we must first look at what electricity actually is.

The word electricity comes from the Greek word "electron" meaning amber because the Greeks established that amber rubbed with fur attracted light objects like feathers. In the 18th century Charles Dufay discovered that there were two kinds of electrical charge. Wax rubbed with a wool cloth shows one kind while glass rubbed with silk shows another. The forces between two of the same charges was repulsion where as between different charges was attraction. When two types were combined they tended to neutralise each other. Benjamin Franklin later called them positive and negative. As discussed before the body has a certain amount of electrical energy which seems to be more prevalent in people with mental illness. The energy is generated by a similar way to the rubbing of a wool cloth with wax or glass with silk in that it is generated through rubbing of the sexual organs (genitals).

These forces have already been discovered in eastern nations and are known as the Yin and Yang. They are as follows =

YIN = SUBMISSIVE, DARK, ABSORBING, EARTH

YANG = DOMINANT, LIGHT, PENETRATING, HEAVEN

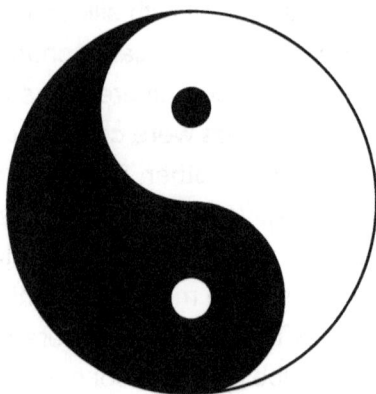

Yin Yang symbol

Because a mental man is more prone to these forces, if he indulges in submissive thoughts he will generate a negative energy which could last for 3 days. This will generate a feeling of being uncomfortable but nothing else unless your bowl has decided it is. If you want to remain feeling comfortable about yourself then you mustn't indulge in any submissive thoughts. It may take a few days for the yang energy to be generated and it seems any submissive thought during masturbation even if only for 5 seconds could disrupt your flow. I remember I was once having sex with a lady and she started to boss me around while we were doing it so I had to stop because I could feel a disruption in my energy. I have concluded the following for the mental man –

Sexual Submission = negative energy = feeling uncomfortable = guilt (anal debating)

Sexual Dominance = positive energy = feeling comfortable = love (if you find it)

Before dismissing any of my theories it's important that the mental man at the very least gives it a try over a period of 3 months. The theory will also work best if you're not taking very strong medication. It's also important that if the man were to masturbate he always has a picture of a woman in front of him rather than getting lost in imagination. While you walk around feeling uncomfortable the mental woman sits and waits for the affection she so desperately needs.

Didn't Frank Sinatra once say "what is a man, what has he got, if not himself then he has not, to say the things he truly feels and not the words of one who kneels". It could be you already have knelt, if this is the case, you could always stand up.

8 Artificial Flavourings / Drugs

The cake will still be formed regardless of whether or not you put any flavouring in to the mixture because the flour used is self raising. In other words flavourings are optional. Artificial flavourings in the mental person are drugs or too much alcohol. There's nothing wrong with drinking alcohol as long as you find a level you're comfortable with, I only drink occasionally for example. Drugs of any kind should be eliminated and cigarettes too. Cigarettes are full of chemicals and also interfere with the mind's well being (the mental persons mind). We will now take a closer look at a few individual drugs to see how they can affect your mind.

Cigarettes – Tobacco traces its history back to the ancient Mayan civilization of America where the tobacco would be chewed, eaten or smoked. The Aztecs later adopted this custom and so did the native American Indians who used smoking in their religious ceremonies. After Christopher Columbus arrived in 1492 he brought tobacco to Europe where people later adopter the practice.

Today, cigarettes contain more than 4000 chemicals. One of the chemicals known as nicotine won't cause cancer however it is responsible for making the cigarette more addictive. Nicotine is as addictive as heroin and cocaine. Some of the affects of smoking include making your skin age faster and staining teeth. Men who smoke are more likely to suffer from impotence. Smoking increases the onset of Type 2 diabetes, heart disease, strokes, blood clots and angina. Breathing problems are caused leaving people breathless and exhausted. All kinds of cancers are caused including mouth, bladder, kidney, stomach, liver etc and there is a higher risk of developing leukaemia. I personally found smoking affected my mental health by reducing my concentration span, reducing my memory and increasing anxiety.

Alcohol - Although it is legal it still remains one of the most dangerous of recreational drugs and can contribute to social, physical and mental problems. Alcohol is classified as a depressant which is the group of drugs that slows the activity in the central nervous system. This interferes with a person's inhibitions, judgement, concentration and motor activity (muscular movement or the nerves surrounding it). The chemical ethyl alcohol is present in all alcoholic drinks and is quickly absorbed into the blood through the lining of the stomach and the intestine. When the ethyl alcohol enters the bloodstream it then affects the central nervous system and binds together certain neurons (nerve cells). One group of neurons affected is the neurotransmitter

GABA. Once this neurotransmitter has been affected a person's inhibitions are interfered with and the individual will become more relaxed. When more alcohol is consumed other areas of the brain are affected resulting in a change of judgment, concentration and speech.

The affects of the alcohol are reduced or disappear when the alcohol concentration in the blood falls. The liver is primarily responsible for breaking down the alcohol and turning it into carbon dioxide and water which is then released by the body. Alcohol abuse varies among people; generally however the person will drink large quantities on a regular basis. They become dependant on the drink to help them through their everyday life however this usually interferes with and has disastrous implications on their work and social lives. Alcohol is responsible for a large number of automobile accidents, rapes, assaults, accidental death and suicide. Physical health problems include liver, heart and immune system damage. Women who drink during pregnancy may provoke "foetal alcohol syndrome" giving the child a range of problems including head and face abnormalities and heart defects. Finally 'Korsakoffs syndrome' is an alcohol related disease which causes mental problems like extreme confusion and memory loss.

Cannabis – A class of drugs taken from a plant known as Cannabis Sativa typically found in warm climates. The most powerful type is known as hashish and the weakest is known as marijuana in the form of crushed leaves and flowering tops of the plant. Cannabis has a long history and was used by the Chinese medical profession 2000 years ago as an anaesthetic. In other countries it was also used for medical purposes like curing insomnia and muscle pain. Marijuana was still being prescribed by doctors in the United States in the early 20th century however as better drugs were being developed it was no longer used. Marijuana then began to be used for recreational use and became an illegal substance.

When taken for recreational use it can produce hallucinogenic, depressant and stimulant affects. Some users will become relaxed and feel more sociable however to others it could provoke the opposite affect. THC (the active ingredient in marijuana) affects the nerve cells in the part of the brain where memories are formed. Because people with mental illness have an adverse disposition to marijuana, a number of reactions are caused. These include a distorted perception of reality, difficulty thinking and problem solving, increased heart rate, anxiety, panic attacks and even suicidal thinking. The level of THC is a lot higher than the marijuana smoked in the 1960's so it really should be avoided.

Amphetamine – A group of drugs described as a stimulant, produced in the laboratory. They were invented in the 1930's by the medical profession in order to treat asthma. The drug soon became know for its stimulant affect and was used by soldiers, truck drivers and pilots who needed help in staying awake. For recreational use it is also taken as a stimulant by all night party goers and some use it to help them stay awake in their day to day work lives. When a user becomes addicted and stops taking the drug depression usually follows. People have been admitted to mental health wards and sectioned whilst under the use of the drug.

Ecstasy - (MDMA) was invented in 1913 by the German chemical company Merck. Ecstasy falls into a category of drugs known as hallucinogens which also includes LSD. The drug affects people by producing illusions, hallucinations and also helps them to stay awake during a party. Ecstasy works by releasing the neurotransmitter dopamine and serotonin simultaneously in various regions of the brain. When the user takes the drug for the very first time the level of serotonin released is quite high and results in a feeling of well being. As the user becomes used to it, the desired effect is achieved by increasing the dose. Ecstasy can produce liver damage and some people have died taking the drug. Another problem with Ecstasy is that the neurotransmitters in the brain become permanently damaged. The brain will only be able to produce a low level of serotonin which can increase mental health problems like ability to concentrate and memory. The drug like most others has contributed towards severe mental health problems leading to hospitalisation.

LSD – is the most powerful of the hallucinogens and was invented by the chemist Albert Hoffman in the 1930's. LSD became popular for recreational use during the 1960's and was used by millions on the party scene. When a person takes this drug the effects are noticed within two hours and the mind enters a state known as hallucinosis. The user may begin to see things that don't exist, objects become distorted or appear to change shape and colours become brighter. Other senses become affected so one might hear things that aren't actually there or become unable to differentiate between hot and cold. LSD is so powerful that even a small dose can produce a hallucination. This drug like others has increased mental health problems.

Cocaine – Classified as a stimulant, one of a group of drugs that increase the activity in the central nervous system. Cocaine is derived from the coca plant usually found in South America. The indigenous people of South America had been chewing the leaves for centuries as it increased energy levels and made people more alert. The drug was first taken from the plant in the 19th century and is described as an unscented, white fluffy powder. Cocaine is usually taken by snorting it through the nose and it is then absorbed by the mucous membrane. Other methods of taking the drug include injecting and smoking.

Free basing is a technique where the pure element of cocaine called alkaloid is chemically separated from the processed cocaine. It is then placed into a special pipe and vaporized by the heat of a flame whilst being inhaled. The most common form of free base cocaine is crack which looks like small crystal rocks.

When taken the drug produces a sudden feeling of well-being and confidence. If a high dose is taken the effect could be similar to that experienced by heroin. The user will begin to feel more talkative, motivated, energetic and excited. The central nervous system is affected because cocaine increases the supply of the neurotransmitter dopamine in areas throughout the brain. Other neurotransmitters affected include norepinephrine and serotonin which also contribute to the affects of the drug. After the user has finished taking the drug and the effects begin to disappear the user may go through a stage of depression and headaches lasting for 24 hours. One of the biggest problems with taking cocaine is overdose which can result in death. Women who use the drug risk having children with abnormalities and are more likely to miscarry. Regular users see their social, family and work relationships ruined. Other problems include memory lose, depression, insomnia and increased anxiety. Some users become confused and their mental health is affected contributing to hallucinations, delusions and psychosis.

Heroin – is one of the most addictive drugs and comes from the sap of the opium poppy. Opium has been used by the medical profession for centuries as it is able to reduce physical and emotional suffering. One of the disadvantages however was its addictiveness. In the 19th century a new substance called morphine was discovered which also came from opium. This drug was even more affective than opium at relieving pain however it also proved to be addictive. During the American civil war of 1861 many soldiers were given morphine when wounded in battle and many became addicted.

At the end of the 19th century Heroin was developed and at the time was considered revolutionary by the medical profession, it was even used as a cough medicine however it later proved to be more addictive than morphine. By the early 20th century the United States government decided to make it illegal with the exception of medical purposes. All drugs taken from opium whether natural or synthetic are characterized as narcotics. There are different methods of taking narcotics which include smoking, inhaling, snorting and injecting. Heroin is usually injected which results in a sudden feeling of well being. This usually follows a pleasant feeling referred to as a "high or nod". During this period the user feels relaxed, happy and care free.

The effects of heroin are created when the drug depresses the central nervous system. Heroin affects receptors that usually receive the neurotransmitters called endorphins which help to relieve pain and emotional tension. This result in the pleasurable feelings associated with taking the drug. The problem with heroin is that when the individual becomes addicted he finds the several hours of high are no longer achieved with a small dose. He will then need to increase the dose and as the body becomes used to the drug the several hours of high are reduced to only one. Eventually he will need to take the drug only to stop the withdrawal symptoms and may turn to criminal activity to feed his habit. Withdrawal symptoms include anxiety, restlessness, sweating, severe twitching, rapid breathing, vomiting, fever, aches, loss of appetite and high blood pressure. During the withdrawal stage an addict may take the same level dose he was on before he went into withdrawal and this can result in an overdose causing death. Drug traffickers often mix heroin with cheaper substitutes and have even been known to mix it with the deadly substance cyanide. Non sterile needles result in a high level of HIV and other infections among heroin users.

During my first episode of mental illness I was a user of marijuana and thought this was the root cause of my illness, it would leave me feeling drained so I decided anything which could be affecting my mental health should stop. There was a point in my life when I deeply regretted ever having taken this drug. I used to think if I could start all over again I wouldn't go near drugs because they caused my mental illness. In hindsight I can firmly conclude that marijuana was not the root cause of my illness though it certainly did exacerbate my condition immensely.

I'm absolutely baffled when I meet someone with mental illness who is still smoking a joint or taking other drugs. You're not a child and there really is no excuse. If you're someone with mental problems then drugs or too much alcohol can only worsen your condition. Different things affect different people differently. Just because your friends do it doesn't necessarily mean you can.

There's lots of help available to stop smoking and taking drugs. I used special gums which release a certain amount of nicotine into the blood stream. Marijuana fuels ignorance so when you have an eventual psychosis your detachment from reality will be far greater and probably of mystic origin. You should try to fill your mind with information and knowledge rather than feeding it drugs.

COOKING PROCESS

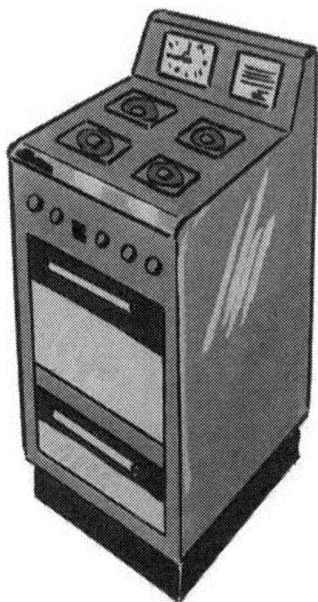

9 Psychosis

Now the cake is complete. The schizophrenia has taken affect. What shall we do with our cake? It's far too big for mum and dad to handle. Oh look there, along comes Miss Curious the psychologist "Can I try some". "Mmmmmmmmm this cake is really really nice I wonder how it's made. I've never had a cake this nice before I wonder what the secret ingredient is! Cake; tell me your secret ingredient. I've never tasted one so nice before, tell me your secret!"

Oh look, along comes Mr Observation the neurologist "can I try some cake? I like the taste but the texture is marvellous. I wonder why it's different to other cakes! I had better put it under the microscope and analyse its genetic make up, or better still run it under the MRI machine to find its secret component."

Then along come the mob "this cake is crap, smells crap too, it's a joke. I know, why don't we rip it apart and have a food fight, its fun" and finally the cake is gone. The cake is gone everybody had a bit to eat and there's nothing left, it's disappeared in to oblivion. But there is something left.........THE BOWL.

If you're someone who has got mental problems then you really are stuck with your bowl. Just because you have a bowl doesn't necessarily mean you have to use it. I have a bowl and I've decided to minimise my stress so there won't be enough butter to make the cake. I've decided to be aware of my stress levels and how they affect me so there won't be any sugar (IBS) in the cake. I have a bowl and I've decided not to add any eggs and flour (sexual negativity). I have a bowl and won't be using any artificial flavouring (drugs). I have a bowl and I'm fed up of cooking.

People will argue that society needs a framework or some kind of ideology in order to function. If this is the case I'm asking people to be more aware of how much their ideals can affect others. What I'm against is when people perceive their ideal as being the best. I live in a democratic, dog eat dog industrialised society and my life has turned upside down and others commit suicide by the thousands. This means that something in a capitalist democracy isn't working and I'm just asking people to acknowledge that just because it works for you, doesn't necessarily mean it works for someone else. Everybody accepts that different foods, drinks and drugs affect different people differently. Why can't they accept that so do their ideals and environments? Some people need a spiritual environment, others like to be in touch with nature, some need less stressful environments and the list goes on.

Even a secular industrialised society has turned in to a religion without realising it. The DSM book of psychiatry is a book full of diagnosis for people who don't fit in to the capitalist machine. In order to give the book credibility another fantasy has been invented the "chemical imbalance or genetic cause". It has become the "psychiatric bible" and if you don't fit in to an industrial dog eat dog environment you are judged by the DSM and doctor just as you are judged by the priest and the bible if you don't fit in to a religious environment. All I'm asking is for people to be less rigid in their ideologies.

The idea of "The Cake Theory" is that one day when a person starts to feel like they don't fit in to society rather than saying "I'm not normal" they say "my environment isn't working for me" and instead of saying "what happening to me?" they say "it must be my involuntary nervous system".

The problem with the psychiatric profession is that they seem to think a chemical imbalance occurs for no apparent reason. For example if somebody gets over worked and is mistreated in the work place they may become depressed and withdrawn. When a person becomes depressed there may be chemical changes going on in the brain. The shocking thing about the psychiatric profession is that they don't explain to the patient how being mistreated and overworked can affect you. The psychiatrist assumes the chemical imbalance took place out of the blue for no apparent reason, which is a travesty.

As we saw in the anthropology section at the start of the theory, the Napoleonic code of 1804 saw the expulsion of religion from institutions replaced by "common sense". Perhaps one day we shall see the psychiatric religion replaced by "understanding".

In the current social climate in the UK there doesn't seem to be an avenue to take for someone who has susceptibility for developing mental health problems. It's important to remember that chronic mental illness could be avoided if measures were put into place. Ideally more emphasis on how stress affects people could be taught at schools from the age of 14. More information on what biochemical reactions caused by stress actually are could be given not in a booklet but by a teacher explaining it to the class. Children could be shown different case studies and also shown what kind of stress people face in other countries. I had no idea what irritable bowel syndrome or migraines were at the age of 25 for example.

I would personally go further by dividing children in to two distinct groups before they go to secondary school. At the moment some schools are divided on the basis of gender, religion, academic ability and even social status. In order to improve mental health I would divide them on personality traits. There could be a secondary school for extroverted children and one for the more introverted. In this scenario the introvert is far more likely to open up rather than feeling intimidated and becoming withdrawn. In the scenario of bullying occurring in an introverted school the bully will simply be removed from the school and sent to the extroverted school.

I must also add most of the knowledge I gained in my life was neither from school nor from university but in my spare time at home. I would make history compulsory because this keeps an individual in touch with reality. Mathematics could be made optional. I felt mathematics only made me confused and didn't help me to understand the world we live in. Young people don't need a pretty academic certificate; they need to feel like they have a place in the community.

Even with measures like the above put in place there will still be people who will find the whole experience of finding a job after they leave school very stressful. When I had my first breakdown at the age of 18 I was told by the medical profession to forget about it and get on with my life, as if nothing had happened. This really is irresponsible; surely a sensible person looks closely at the past in order to stop it from happening in the future. The doctors wrote in my medical records that my initial breakdown was caused by stress. If that was the case why send me back in to the rat race knowing that my chances of relapse and developing chronic mental illness were enormous considering I had a breakdown at such a young age? It's a bit like curing someone from the flu and then sending them to the North Pole wearing only a T Shirt, jeans and armed with some medication in their back pocket. The medical profession doesn't seem to have a problem spending money on patients when their illness is chronic so why not invest more time in helping someone on their very first breakdown. In my case I found the whole experience of looking for a job extremely stressful. I would have liked to work part time in a library or museum in an environment I find relaxing. Considering these institutions are run by the state and the doctors are paid by the state it would have been helpful if the state could have helped me in finding a job.

Another measure to implement could be to characterize jobs in terms of stress levels. For example a very stressful job will be given a 5 and a low stress level job would be given a 1. The jobs which are least stressful could be available exclusively to those who find stressful environments devastating.

Some people thrive on stress, the more they get the more they want, however some people like myself find they can't handle it. It's important to remember I'm not someone who has decided to take the easy way out. If I could handle stress I would gladly work 12 hour days. However if this doesn't work for me why do I have to be pressured to the point of losing my sanity and possibly developing chronic mental illness? Then people have the audacity to turn around and say "It's an illness that happens like cancer and we don't know why".

The irony is of course that some 6000 years ago the early Egyptians were probably right. Mental illness is very much relative to your surrounding environment. To think today some people still believe that mental illness is a punishment from God. But do you really think God is someone who would inflict so much pain and suffering on to a person?

In reality the root cause of mental illness is people's inability to respect and care for one another. If people were more considerate to those who are easily stressed or upset there wouldn't be a problem.

These so called 'secure people' could argue that if my environment isn't working for me I should leave the country and find one that does. I would say in reply "Why don't you leave the country seeing you're the cause of my problem? And while you're at it, take your stupid dream of being successful and better than others with you."

Some doctors believe there is a gene which causes mental illness. I don't think there is a gene which causes mental illness although there may be a genetic cause for some people being unable to handle too much stress. However I don't believe this to be the case either because as we saw in the stress section of the theory different environments affect different people differently which contradicts the genetic argument. I was wondering if there was a gene which made people confident and inconsiderate. Is there a genetic cause for a businessman being unable to function in a left wing society? Is there a genetic cause for women being materialistic? What kind of a man joins the armed forces? Does a soldier have a genetic cause for wanting to kill a fellow human being? Let us take the current situation in Iraq for example.

Iraq used to be called Mesopotamia and was the home of great civilisations like Babylon and Assyria which was later invaded by the Persians. It was then invaded by Arabs who introduced Islam. The Mongols invaded in 1258 and the Turkish Ottoman Empire invaded in the 16th century. Britain invaded the area in 1916 and renamed the country Iraq and today the American's have decided to invade.

The only logical explanation for the above is that a specific group of people must have a genetic cause for making them want to invade and kill fellow human beings. Could we possibly genetically modify babies so these people no longer exist in the future?

The mob now seems to be dividing its self in to two distinct categories like children in a playground. On the one side we have the Muslims with their head scarf saying "look at me, I believe and have lots of faith". On the other side we have the Christians with their wooden Cross saying "Yes but look at my Cross it's so big and full of faith na na nanana". At the bottom we have the mental person who couldn't care less about who is better or worse but would just like to be equal.

So who then is this man of mystery they call Mr. Schizophrenia. In many respects he's like a snail. He has no need for superficial trivia, a man who needs love and affection. So why then does he remain in his shell? Is it because he wasn't loved as a child? Is it because he has a chemical imbalance? Is there something wrong in the shells construction preventing him to leave? Or maybe every time he comes out of his shell he is unable to see it. But could he if he really looked hard enough?

Having come to these conclusions I ask myself "Why on earth did I want to be friends with such a horrible group of people back at school". Then my heart burns and says "look what these Mother F***ers have done to me, look at what people have turned me into, why don't they F*** themselves." But then I turn on the TV and watch the News "ha hahahaaa they already have."

www.ingramcontent.com/pod-product-compliance
Lightning Source LLC
Chambersburg PA
CBHW031217270326
41931CB00006B/592